INTERMITTENT FASTING 16:8

A Complete Guide for Weight Loss with Delicious Meal Plan and Recipes to Easily Follow the Intermittent Fasting Method 16:8.

SABRINA SMERALDINI

@ Copyright di Sabrina Smeraldini

www.italianstylerecipe.net

Disclaimer

All rights reserved. No part of this book may be reproduced by any mechanical, photographic, or electronic process, or in the form of a phonographic recording; nor may it be stored in a retrieval system, transmitted, or otherwise be copied for public or private use—other than for "fair use" as brief quotations embodied in articles and reviews—without prior written permission of the publisher.

The author of this book does not dispense medical advice or prescribe the use of any technique as a form of treatment for physical, emotional, or medical problems without the advice of a physician, either directly or indirectly. The intent of the author is only to offer information of a general nature to help you in your quest for well-being. In the event you use any of the information in this book for yourself, the author and the publisher assume no responsibility for your actions.

@ Copyright di Sabrina Smeraldini

http://www.italianstylerecipe.net/

TABLE OF CONTENTS

Introduction 1

    1. 1

    Healthy & Tasty 1

    2. 4

    The Body Needs Nutrients 4

    3. 6

    Keep The Body Strong 6

    4. 10

    Keep The Goal in Mind 10

Part I - Intermittent Fasting Overview 12

    1. 12

    Intermittent Fasting: The Basics 12

    2. 15

    Intermittent Fasting: Various Formulas (Brief Explanation Of The Fasting Methods) 15

    3. 20

    Intermittent Fasting: How & Why It Works 20

    4. 23

Intermittent Fasting: Benefits And Downsides (Who Is It For?) 23

5..26

Fasting: Science & History (Some Research) 26

Intermittent Fasting 16:8 28

1..28

What Is The 16:8 Method? 28

2..30

16:8 Method for Beginners 30

3..32

Benefits & Side Effects Of 16:8 Fasting (Workout: yes or no?) 32

Part III - Intermittent Fasting 16:8 Step by Step Guide 39

1..39

16:8 Method: How to Follow It 39

2..48

Intermittent Fasting Delicious Meal Plan 48

3..59

Adequate Hydration 59

4..61

Intermittent Fasting: The Easy Strategy (Extra Info & Tips) 61

Final Thoughts 65

Conclusion 68

About the author 69

INTRODUCTION

1

Healthy & Tasty

The main difference between a common diet and an eating program is that the former is temporary whereas the latter is a lifestyle.

If you say *"I'll start on Monday"* that's a diet, it is usually restrictive and feels like punishment and there are some types of food that are banned. A diet sounds like this: *"I can't eat cookies anymore, I'm on a diet"* or *"Pizza? No thanks. I'm on a diet"* or *"Oh...I wish I could get myself an ice cream but I am on this diet and it's so hard to resist...Ok, ok just this one time and then I'll never cheat again"*

This usually leads to guilt and consequently even more eating. It's a diet!

If you say *"I'd like to feel better in my own skin, feel healthier and more vital"*, then you are looking for a lifestyle change.

A lifestyle change sounds like this: *"Well, I've had a healthy breakfast, lunch was balanced, I gave my body plenty of nutrients. I can have a cookie and it won't make that much difference. Besides I'm planning on eating a light dinner."*

This usually leads to sticking to your healthy eating program, feeling better, losing weight and maintaining your shape.

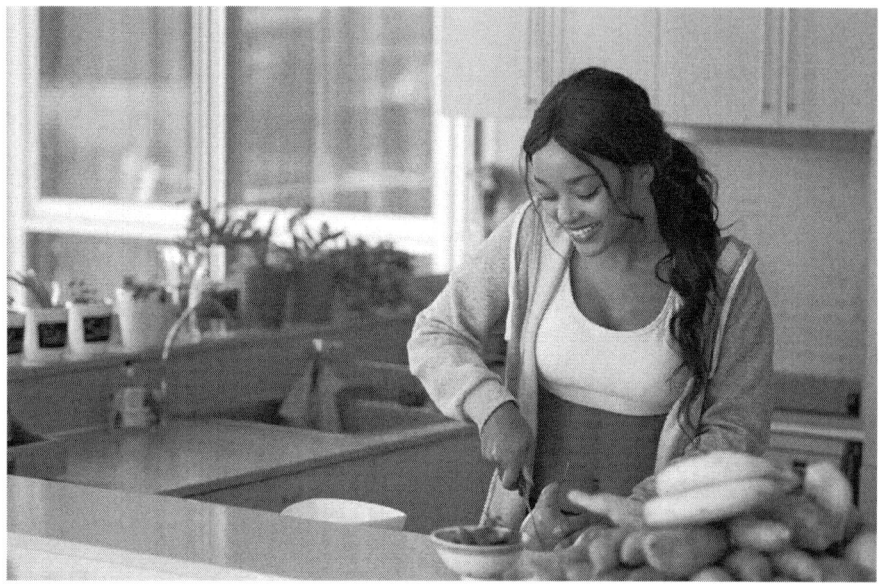

So, as you can deduce now, a healthy eating program doesn't mean that you have to give up taste or your favorite foods. It simply means balance and moderation.

Healthy food doesn't have to be tasteless either. The key is to give your body the nutrients it requires to stay healthy and give you energy. If you choose your favorite healthy ingredients, then you can look around and search for different recipes and prepare those ingredients in many ways.

If your overall eating is balanced and healthy you can allow yourself to have a treat every once in a while. Even among those treats you can choose higher quality ones. Let's give some examples.

Let's say you really like ice-cream. Instead of buying cheap, packaged and filled with chemicals, you can go to a place where they make homemade ice cream with genuine ingredients.

The same goes for cookies, pizza or bread.

The problem is with foods that are not even "real foods" and we could then call them "items" or fake foods. These include industrially made products and beverages that don't even exist in nature. You can recognize those by their color (usually neon colored or very bright anyways) and by the list of ingredients on the package (very long, hard to pronounce or even understand).

When I say the problem, what I mean is that your body doesn't even recognize those foods, it doesn't know what to do with them and so they pollute your body, create imbalances and in the long run they can create illnesses.

Now that we are clear about the difference between an eating program and a diet, that we have recognized that healthy can be tasty, we can say that although it's called *"The Intermittent Fasting Diet"*, it isn't a diet in the most common way in which the word is used. It's more than a diet, it is *a change in lifestyle*.

It's especially called a diet when referred to as the various methods in which you can follow it. More on this later in the book.

Sabrina Smeraldini

2

The Body Needs Nutrients

Just because an eating program is a lifestyle change and not a diet, that doesn't mean that calories don't count. If you follow a healthy eating program you still need to be aware of calories in and calories out, if you want to lose weight.

It's a simple math thing. It's not possible to lose weight if your calorie intake is higher than the calories you burn.

With that said, it's important to notice that your body needs nutrients and if you give it sufficient nutrients it will reward you with enough energy and it won't keep craving for more.

If you consider comfort food as an occasional treat and not the norm you will naturally lower your calorie intake.

By following a healthy eating program, instead of a temporary diet, you will be focusing on high-nutrient foods and you will reduce prepackaged-high-carb-empty-calories and junk food to a minimum.

The solution to a healthier lifestyle is to give your body enough nutrients so that it can function at its fullest.

Think of it this way, in order to do all the wonderful things of daily life, the body needs fuel and nutritious food is that fuel. *Eating is giving energy to your body, not just filling your stomach.* In fact, you can be full and the body could still be starving.

Nutritious foods for the body is food that belongs to the various groups of macronutrients such as healthy carbs and fats, proteins, fiber, vitamins and minerals. The simpler the better. We'll talk about specific foods in more detail later in the book.

3

Keep The Body Strong

Obesity is a huge phenomenon, especially in western countries, and it's still increasing to the point that it is starting to spread to eastern nations as well.

The problem with overweight and obesity goes far deeper than physical appearances. It is a serious issue that may lead to illnesses and in extreme cases to death.

Intermittent Fasting 16:8

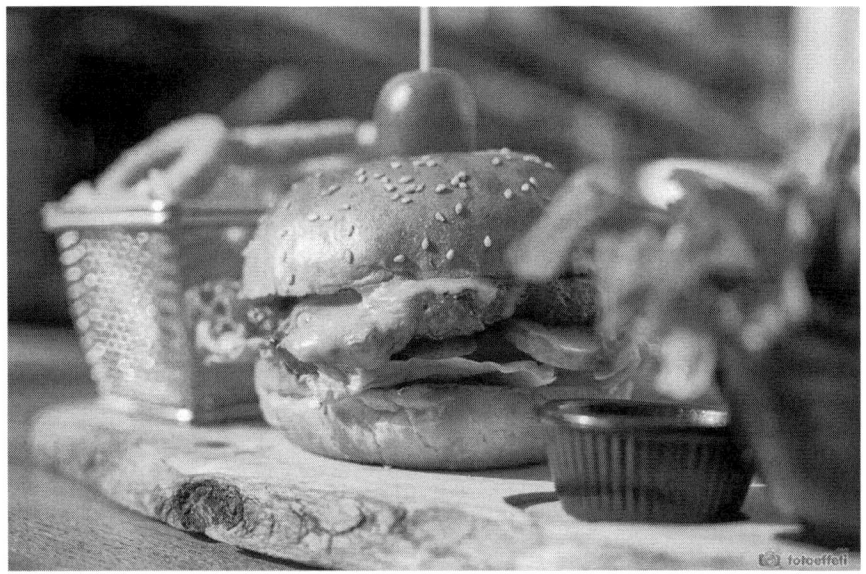

What causes obesity? One might say: overeating. But overeating is an addiction and an addiction is usually a covering up of something deeper. It is usually an emotional problem. They are called *comfort foods* for a reason.

Comfort foods are addictive if you overindulge. But, as I said before, some foods are fake, industrially made and not nature made. These processed foods (or "items") are not recognized by the body and they cause great imbalances.

All these foods cause blood sugar levels to spike and this in turn leads to fat storage and insulin insensitivity.

One might also argue that healthy options are much more expensive but, is that really true in the long term? Being healthy doesn't cost much in terms of prescription drugs and visits to doctors. Actually it costs nothing. Being sick, on the contrary, can be extremely expensive. And that's one thing. The other thing is that I always suggest to choose *quality over quantity*.

You don't have to eat four scoops of ice cream; you can eat two of a higher quality. You don't have to eat a steak every day, it's better to eat a grass-fed quality beef steak once or twice a week.

The same concept applies to all kinds of foods.

By feeding your body with healthy, nutritious foods, by avoiding simple carbs (which is basically sugar in all its many forms), unhealthy fats and fake foods (which is also referred to as empty calorie food because it contains no nutritional value), you are on the right track to achieving amazing results.

Another reason that causes excess weight and in extreme cases obesity, is the kind of lifestyle that one leads. Staying active keeps the body strong and alive. A sedentary lifestyle weakens the body. It all boils down to habits. *But the good news is that you can break a habit.* It takes dedication, consistency, a little time and practice.

One step at a time. You can go for a walk instead of watching another episode of your favorite show. You can eat a fresh apple instead of drinking a bottled apple juice filled with sugar. All those things matter. *Transformation is the result of many little steps taken each day, it is not a quantum leap that you take overnight.*

Working out helps you pick healthier foods. This is because you feel cleaner and better and also because you don't want to ruin all the hard work that you've done by eating badly.

With that said, it is now clear that the combination of leading an active lifestyle and selecting the right foods are the two factors that combined work together to *keep the body strong.*

Intermittent Fasting 16:8

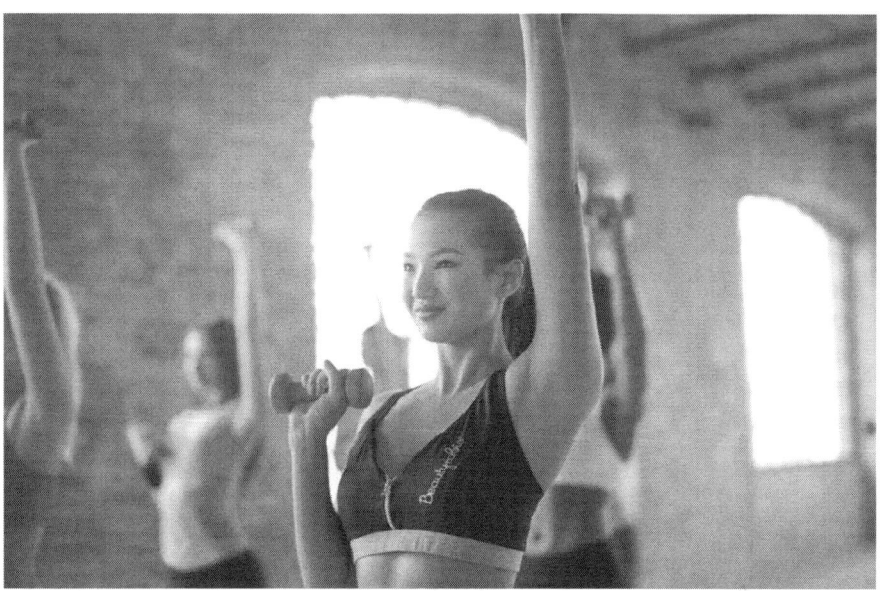

4

Keep The Goal in Mind

At first your body will rebel against the changes in your eating habits so imagine that you have to deal with a child and you are changing some kind of rule. The baby at first will cry a lot and complain but if you stay calm and patient and don't give in, after a short while, the baby will learn and accept the new rule. The same goes for your body. *Treat it with patience but be firm in your decision and keep your goal in mind.*

Since adapting to a new diet is not really the easiest thing, make sure you make a decision and follow through.

In order to do it, it helps to know why you are doing it, *what is your motivation?* It might be as simple as looking good in your skinny jeans or having energy to play with you kids or your dog, staying healthy and vital, preparing for a wedding or a romantic vacation, increasing self-esteem.

Whatever it may be, just make sure you keep the goal in mind. This will help you especially in moments of hunger and when you are feeling sad or discouraged.

It might also help to have a vision board with pictures and inspiring quotes to keep you up with your weight-loss and healthy goals. You could carry a list of the benefits of intermittent fasting (we'll explore them later on in the book), exercising and eating nutritious foods to remind yourself why you are doing it.

If you stick with it, it will get easier.

Part I - Intermittent Fasting Overview

1

Intermittent Fasting: The Basics

Intermittent Fasting is an eating program which requires you to go through phases of eating and not eating. Intermittent fasting, although only relatively recently discovered for weight purposes and health benefits, has been around for many, many years. It is an eating pattern widely used not only by athletes but by all kinds of people including men, women, teens etc.

Most people fast on a daily basis without even realizing it. Just think about the word "breakfast?" It literally means to break the overnight fast.

Since intermittent fasting is considered a method to *cleans* and *detox* the body, it is an option that many people are choosing in order to *improve their general health* and it can also help those who are looking to get into shape and *lose weight*.

The intermittent fasting diet is sometimes called the feast and famine diet. It isn't a new fad, actually it has been around for quite some time. The reason it became really popular is that it worked for many people.

Fasting has been around in one form or another from the beginning of mankind. Recently, it has experienced a reawakening among athletes, gym enthusiasts, and dieters. More and more people are fasting to get rid of toxins, improve their health, and lose excess fat.

Some love its convenience and simplicity. Others feel confused by all the different fasting plans out there.

There are some common questions among dieters like:

What can you eat on fasting days?

What's allowed and what's forbidden?

Is it necessary to track calories?

Do I need to include all macros or exclude carbs?

Should I watch portions, or eat as much as I think I need?

Can I workout if I'm fasting?

Can I avoid working out since I'm on a diet?

In this Guide we are going to answer to these questions and address other topics on dieting as well as try to clear out any confusion about the intermittent fasting diet.

Sabrina Smeraldini

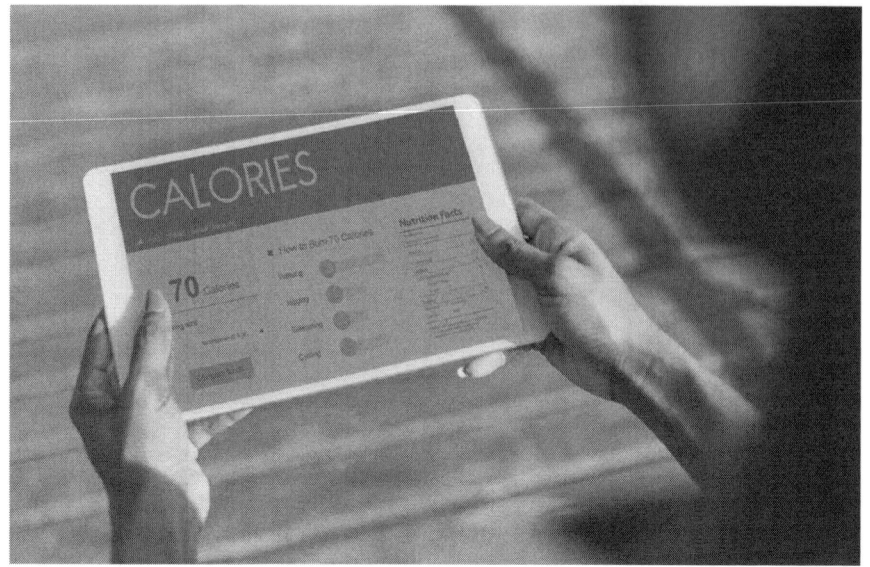

2

Intermittent Fasting: Various Formulas (Brief Explanation Of The Fasting Methods)

There are various different types of the Intermittent Fasting diet. The main difference consists of *when* you eat and *when* you fast.

There is more than one way to fast. Actually, there are multiple types of protocols to choose from in the Intermittent Fasting Regimen. In order to select the right one for you, you need to have a brief overview of the different methods and then *decide according to your own needs* depending on the schedule and other details.

Intermittent fasting mostly changes your eating time schedule since the element that most distinguishes this program from any other diet is *when* you eat.

The 16:8

One of the easiest and most popular method is the 16:8. Easiest because it is the one where you actually fast for a shorter period of time during waking hours.

What happens is that you fast for 16 hours and you can have your meals during the remaining 8 hours. The thing is that most of the fasting period occurs while you sleep which, as you can deduce, makes it even easier to stick to. This type is also called LeanGains and it is one of the simplest among the others.

The goal is to go *16 hours straight* without eating and you can choose this period of time according to your schedule and habits.

Let's say you enjoy eating dinner with your family, you don't want to give that up so you might want to start your 16 hours fast from after dinner until the next day.

Also make sure to keep in mind when are the times of day when you tend to get really hungry and plan accordingly.

Eat-Stop-Eat

Another method is called Eat-Stop-Eat or 24-Hour Fast. This is a bit harder because it requires you to go *24 hours in a row* without eating. That's a full day!

If you opt for this method, you might want to do it once or twice a week. If you've never been on a diet, or if you are just starting out, you might want to begin with one full day of fasting per week.

Remember not to drink your calories! There has to be no calorie intake during those 24-hour period so plain water is the best choice, although you can also have tea or coffee as long as you don't add sugar, milk or cream.

It goes without saying that for the rest of the week it's best to keep your body healthy and vital by making wise food choices. Choose foods that is nutritious and delicious, foods that make you feel good and clean.

To follow this protocol, you can either start in the morning and fast until the next day, but this means you are going past the 24 hours, or you can start sometime at midday for example. And this is what most people prefer.

The Warrior Protocol

This is called "The Warrior" because you need to be a warrior in order to survive a longer fasting period. It is one of the strictest intermittent fasting methods. Actually, the reason why it's called "The Warrior Diet" is that it comes from a Paleo idea of eating like our ancient ancestors who had to go out in the wilderness to hunt and search for foods and only ate when food was available, when they were able to find it or catch it. This is also why it is sometime referred to as "feast and famine program".

To follow this protocol, you eat one large meal and then fast for the next 24 hours.

Another characteristic of The Warrior Method is that you still need to stick to caveman eating habits when you do eat! Kind of like Paleo but not really…Just common sense, ask yourself what would somebody in the wilderness eat? Meat, fish, fruits, vegetables…the simplest things, basic survival foods, nothing fancy!

Just be mindful of the quality of the foods that you choose. When buying meat for example opt for grass fed, choose cage free eggs and poultry, wild caught meat and grass fed butter. This should be the case not only if you are following "The Warrior Methods", but also if you are aiming at an overall healthier lifestyle.

If it's possible, buy local or at a farmer's market. In my experience, I can't imagine not buying these type of products at the market because where I grew up, in Tuscany with my Grandma, it was just the normal thing to do. My Grandma would grow her own vegetables in her garden or we would go together to the market and buy fresh, genuine products. Then we would prepare our meal at home, using those fresh and nutritious ingredients.

If you get the habit of buying these type of products, you'll have an opportunity to enjoy foods, especially meats, that are hormone and chemical free. The benefits on your overall health will be nothing short of amazing.

Alternate Day

Another way to follow the intermittent fasting diet is the Alternate Day. To do it you fast every other day. You can experiment and for example choose the 16:8 method every other day or perhaps a full 24 hours fasting every other day.

Choose what works best for you, according to your schedule and the messages you receive from your body. That means, pay attention to how you feel!

Some people choose to include just water (coffee or tea) during fasting, others include up to 500 calories.

The 5:2

The 5:2 is self-explanatory: you eat for 5 days and fast the other 2 of the week. Again, that doesn't mean that you can eat pasta, bread and pizza for 5 days straight and then fast. Keep it clean and fresh, you can still have a pizza every once in a while, actually you can still have all your favorite foods if you consume it in moderation and if it's of good quality and made with fresh, genuine ingredients.

While the general idea behind the use of intermittent fasting remains the same, there are many variations of intermittent fasting that serve as perfect diet plans for different individuals depending on their personal requirements, preferences and goals.

Before we discuss the most common types of intermittent fasting diets, there are a few things that you need to keep in mind. When you consider adopting any type of intermittent fasting diet, remember that the different types of diets will yield different results. While all of them will provide various benefits in their own way, they will work differently for different people.

When you decide to choose an intermittent fasting diet, *do not force yourself* towards a certain type. If the decision for it does not come easily, it may not be the right option for you. *For any diet to actually work, it is essential that you have a positive mind-set for it.* If you do not want the benefits of the diet to be short-lived, always choose a diet plan that will make your life easier. That means that you want to choose a diet that can fit easily in your lifestyle and can help you towards your goals.

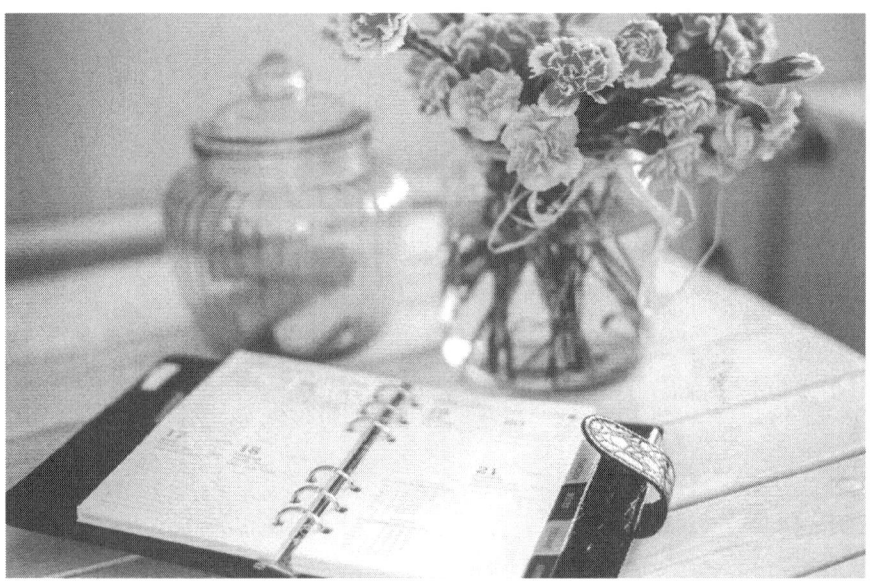

3

Intermittent Fasting: How & Why It Works

In the Intermittent Fasting program, you alternate eating and fasting periods. The fasting is to be considered a period of time in which you give your body a rest and a chance to cleanse itself. It's like a detox. Not eating allows the body to heal and put to use the nutrients that it received.

The fasting also helps to avoid sugar spikes and crashes, your levels of insulin (sugar) will remain more stable. This is a good thing because consequently hunger stabilizes.

During fasting time, the body is going to burn fat. Extra calorie intake turns to fat that get stored in the body, as a "provision". The fasting is for the body to use that "provision" and burn it.

The body tends to burn energy that is immediately available (food you just ate). Unless it has to, it doesn't burn the "provision".

As I've mentioned, the intermittent fasting eating program consists of two phases: eating period and fasting period, *these are also referred to as windows.*

During the eating window, make sure you always have healthy options available. It's harder to resist certain foods when you are hungry and the contrary is also true so it's easy to resist if you are not as hungry. If you always have healthy options available, you are less likely to become really hungry.

As you continue on your healthy eating plan, eventually you'll end the constant hunger and low energy attacks (cravings) that are so common when you are not mindful of your eating habits.

So the idea of intermittent fasting is to follow these healthy guidelines during the eating window and to allow your body to clean up during fasting.

The intermittent fasting program can help you lose weight if you are aware (and therefore if you are able to avoid) of certain misperceptions.

For example, just because you are fasting for a certain period of time, that doesn't mean that you can overeat during the eating window.

Also, if you want to lose weight and feel healthier, you need to choose some kind of physical activity that appeals to you. It doesn't have to be extreme but *you should be moving your body at least 20 minutes almost every day.*

There are so many activities for you to choose from and you could even pick a workout video on YouTube and follow it, if you don't have time to go to the gym. Or, you could run, ride a bike, go for a swim, do some aerobics or Pilates, play tennis. The options are endless.

If you are following the intermittent fasting diet but you are not losing weight it might be that you are drinking your calories and you are not counting those. *Beverages are as important as food.* Many people drink their calories through sugar dense, carbonated sodas which are filled with chemicals and sugar, although some are not aware of that.

If during the eating window you have pancakes for breakfast, cupcakes in the afternoon and pizza for dinner, it doesn't matter if you are fasting, you are not going to lose weight or feel better.

Also, if that is the kind of food that you eat on a regular basis, it will be much harder for you to fast because food that is rich in carbs, simple carbs – like baked products, make you want more of the same.

As for any other things in life, it takes a little while to adjust to a new habit. So at first you might even feel worse than before and feel like you are always hungry. That is because the body is getting rid of all the toxins and – if you don't give up immediately – you will adapt.

Before you start fasting, experiment putting long periods of time between your meals this will help in addition to reducing simple carbs and sugar and increasing protein and fiber (more fruits and vegetables). Start doing this for about 3 weeks before you begin the new program.

4

Intermittent Fasting: Benefits And Downsides (Who Is It For?)

Many people find it hard not to think about food during fasting. This is especially true if you treat it like some sort of punishment and you count the hours for the fasting to be over.

Fasting is not about avoiding food but giving your body a break.

I suggest that you treat fasting as a regenerating time for yourself and for your body. By approaching it in a more positive way it becomes easier to follow it.

Hunger may cause Anger!

Some people become very irritable when they are hungry. And this is a downside. The body likes routines and if you don't give it sufficient food at the appointed time you may notice that even a trivial matter can cause anger or irritation.

You could use this opportunity as a spiritual practice to become more aware of your feelings and their cause. Start paying more attention to your inner state. After a while, as we've already mentioned, the body adapts to the new schedule. Also, listening to music and walking outside really helps in this case.

Initially, fasting can also cause headaches and fatigue. These are usually the symptoms of hypoglycemia, which is essentially a sugar deficiency in the blood stream.

This condition is particularly likely to happen to people addicted to certain foods which are filled with fats and sugar. Your body will need time to adapt to the energy crashes and even though reverting to snacks can be tempting, because you experience cravings, recognize that it's an addiction – a sugar addiction - so if you give in, if you don't break the habit, you remain addicted.

Since fasting reduces the blood sugar, intermittent fasting is not recommended for those with low blood sugar or those who have been diagnosed with diabetes. Therefore, *it is necessary that you take advice from your doctor before you decide to incorporate intermittent fasting into your lifestyle.*

One of the greatest advantages of the intermittent fasting program is its *simplicity*. As long as you know the basics of healthy nutrition such as the main nutrient groups (protein, fiber, healthy fats, vitamins and minerals and different types of carbs), and how different foods have different effects on the body, you simply need to schedule and plan and keep up the initial enthusiasm.

With intermittent fasting, you are more likely to learn to eat better overall.

When it comes to weight-loss, of course calorie counting matters. Research showed that, on average, participants of the intermittent fasting diet ate at least 350 calories less per day than if they were not following this plan. When you only have an eight or 10-hour feeding window, you may not be able to eat as much food as usual. This automatically limits your total calorie intake, leading to fat loss.

Find out how many calories you need to maintain the weight you want to be and stick to that caloric level.

Other benefits of this regimen include improved cardiovascular function, stronger immune system and decreased blood pressure.

When the intermittent fasting diet is followed correctly, it regulates your appetite and keeps hunger at bay.

However, intermittent fasting is not considered a good idea for someone who is underweight. For that you can consider following the *Mediterranean Diet* for example which is considered to be one of the healthiest diet ever.

I've written an entire collection of books on The Mediterranean Diet so I'm not going in more details here.

Intermittent Fasting is NOT good for you if…

Intermittent fasting is not good for you've tried it and you continue to feel sick even after a short period of adjustment.

Some people have low blood sugar and other conditions that may not allow them to fast. If you're feeling dizzy, weak, or just plain sick, break the fast and eat something nutritious.

Listen to your body and proceed accordingly. It's normal to experience fatigue and headaches at the beginning, but these symptoms should go away within a short time.

Intermittent fasting is probably not good for you if you have a medical condition. Always consult your doctor before starting a diet or an exercise program.

If you have diabetes do not use this plan unless you get your doctor's permission. This type of plan will impact your blood sugar and if you have an imbalance due to diabetes it could be detrimental to your health.

Whether you do have any type of medical condition or not, always consult with your doctor first.

5

Fasting: Science & History (Some Research)

The origin of the intermittent fasting diet goes back to the way our ancestors ate. At that time, food was not around the corner. No fridge, no electricity, no fast food restaurants, no cars and no drive thru. If you wanted to eat, you had to grow your fruits and vegetables, hunt, go fishing somewhere. The result is that food was not only scarce (not available every day, and this is the idea behind fasting) but also very simple. No processed, no packaged, no chemicals.

Simply cooked, perhaps directly on fire, maybe a little salt…I would add some extra virgin olive oil to that as well. (Of course I would, I'm Italian. But it's good for you!).

On days when you managed to have food through hunting, fishing or a good harvest, you would have had a feast. If, on the contrary, the pickings were slim and there was no food, you'd go hungry. The only difference between this and the intermittent fasting diet is that in the past you had no choice.

Because of this manner of eating and fasting, and because food was very simple and genuine, our ancestors were not overweight. They didn't know anything about obesity. Also, please notice that going hunting, fishing and growing vegetables is to be considered our ancestor's version of gym activities.

Intermittent fasting has been subject to extensive research. Some studies on this subject were performed at the Laboratory of Neurosciences at the National Institute of Aging.

The results of these many studies on intermittent fasting showed that it can have a positive effect on your cognitive health as well. This means that it may improve brain and memory health. Consequently, it can reduce the risk of contracting brain-related illnesses like dementia and Alzheimer.

This dietary plan improves insulin sensitivity, boosts metabolism, and keeps your heart healthy. It also causes your body to burn stored fat for fuel instead of glucose.

Besides reducing hunger, improving mental focus, and lowering blood glucose levels, cycling between periods of fasting and eating can preserve muscle strength and torch fat. Compared to other weight loss methods, it doesn't cause muscle loss. Most athletes who apply intermittent fasting, experience greater energy and strength, improved concentration, and enhanced performance.

By reducing blood sugar and insulin levels, following the intermittent diet plan helps in keeping your energy steady throughout the day. It also lowers LDL cholesterol, which is the bad kind, and raises HDL, which is the good kind. This consequently helps reduce heart disease risk.

INTERMITTENT FASTING 16:8

1

What Is The 16:8 Method?

The 16:8 methods consists of a fasting window of 16 hours and an eating window of 8 hours.

If you eat dinner at 7.00 p.m. and eat breakfast at 11.00 a.m. the next day, you've been fasting for 16 hours.

Let's explore a bit more. If you have an 8-hour eating window and a 16-hour fasting window, you will need to consume all your calories for the day during the 8 hours. In the example above that would mean between 11.00 a.m. and 7.00 p.m.

This is why I personally find the 16:8 method to be the best solution to follow the intermittent fasting diet. It's very close to what is considered "the norm" and therefore, pretty easy to follow and stick with it without starving, feeling deprived or experiencing fatigue and loss of energy.

Intermittent Fasting 16:8

The 16:8 is sometimes referred to as the LeanGains diet. It consists of fasting for 16 hours (women might choose 14 hours) and eating regularly during the remaining 6 or 8 hours.

This fasting plan is one of the most followed because it can easily be incorporated into any lifestyle.

I find that usually the simple things are the ones that work best. If you have to start following complex schemes, carbohydrate strategies, charts, endless lists and weird ingredients to incorporate to your meal then it's much easier to give up after a short period of time.

What it takes however is motivation and self-discipline and those come naturally when you are clear about why you are doing what you are doing. If you have a purpose you can tolerate a little discomfort. If you don't have a purpose, no amount of will power will ever be enough.

2

16:8 Method for Beginners

If long periods of fasting scare you, if 24 hours seems like a very long time for you to fast, you could choose to start by trying the 16-hour fast. This is considered one of the easiest even more so because about half of the 16 hours are spent sleeping.

If you follow this type of Intermittent Fasting program, which is the 16:8 method, you have an eating window of eight hours.

The eating period should be ideally around midday so that your body is not processing insulin when you sleep. However, when you are starting out try different ways to assess their impact on your routine and body. If it is causing you too much stress and discomfort, it's time to reassess your diet plan, take a deep breath and try a different way.

Try to avoid stress as much as possible by practicing present moment awareness. This is really important because stress is a toxic emotion and the whole point about fasting it to give your body a rest and a chance to cleanse itself. You create stress for yourself when you start thinking about the million things you have to do and all the problems that need to be solved. Keep in mind though that you can only ever do one thing at a time in this present moment.

Let's now take a look at the most important guideline about the eating window. Avoid anything that's junk food or packed with empty calories as much as possible. This will safeguard your overall health. Make sure you get in your fruit and vegetables, but don't be afraid to give yourself a treat every now and then (moderation is key).

Another thing that helps, especially if you want to lose weight, is to eat the last meal of the day early and not eat anything before going to bed. In addition, delay your breakfast. Give yourself some time in the morning before you eat your first meal of the day.

Make sure you are aware of the calorie intake and you could treat it like a budget. Try it as an experiment. Let's say you can take in up to 2,000 calories per day: That's it. That is your calorie budget for the day. You could spend it all at once (I doubt it) or you can spread it throughout the day. You could eat one single thing that has 2,000 calories in it (I doubt it) or you can pick a variety of different foods and follow a more balanced program, the 16:8 for instance.

At the beginning it might be harder. Build up the new habits gradually by decreasing your calorie intake and adding some exercise activity. Give your body time to adapt to the new regimen and be patient with yourself. If you beat yourself up, then you'll start feeling guilty and chances are that you are going to give the whole thing up. The body has the ability to adapt.

3

Benefits & Side Effects Of 16:8 Fasting (Workout: yes or no?)

The best advantage of the 16:8 method is that your body will not go into starvation mode because you will be eating and consuming calories during waking hours.

You can actually drink lots of water as soon as you wake up; have a fresh fruit platter for breakfast at 11.00 a.m. then a salad and some protein for lunch; a small snack (like a handful of nuts for example) in the afternoon and a light dinner around 6.30 – 7.00 p.m.

During the 16-hour window your body will start using the insulin and fat for energy. It doesn't matter if you're awake or sleeping; your body will still be burning calories for all the different bodily processes such as repair and maintenance. These calories will be coming from your stored fats. This is what makes the intermittent fasting 16:8 an effective weight-loss program.

Intermittent fasting has various health benefits and probably that is one of the reasons why it is growing in popularity.

One of the benefits of the intermittent fasting diet is that it reduces hunger and cravings.

When produced in excess, the hunger hormone ghrelin causes you to eat more. After a few days of intermittent fasting, your ghrelin and leptin levels return to normal. Higher leptin levels, on the other hand, curb hunger and cravings. These hormones play a major role in weight-loss. Intermittent fasting regulates leptin and ghrelin production, which, in turn, reduces hunger and promotes satiety.

Although it is probably mainly followed for weight-loss purposes, the intermittent fasting diet has a much broader list of benefits.

Following the latest fad, instead of sticking to a healthy regimen, is not only useless for weight-loss purposes, it can actually be harmful for the body. Too many changes in short periods of time can lead to various issues with digestion, weight gain, and abdominal pain.

I suggest that you focus on feeling good and eating healthy without feeling deprived. That means that you may want to experiment with different methods and then decide what works for you. The reason why so many people are having success with the intermittent fasting program is that it is flexible (as we've seen you can decide among various types of plan) and simple enough.

Another important benefit of intermittent fasting is that it can help control sugar levels in the blood. This is essential because sugar spikes and crashes is the main cause of cravings.

When you follow intermittent fasting appropriately over a prolonged period of time, you start increasing insulin resistance and lowering blood glucose levels naturally.

Even though some people say that you can eat whatever you want during the eating window, being on some sort of program to lose weight - or increase your health - requires you to be mindful of what you eat and it leads to making healthier choices. This is another benefit of choosing the intermittent fasting diet.

Eating nutrient dense foods, as opposed to junk food and empty calories, generates amazing benefits for your weight, heart health, cholesterol, even bone structure.

While intermittent fasting can be a great tool to help you lose weight, control your eating, and learn healthier patterns with food and workouts, *there are some side effects to consider.*

Now that we've seen the benefits let's take a look at what are considered to be the downsides. Let's briefly go through the side effects of the intermittent fasting diet.

One of the potential drawbacks to intermittent fasting has to do with the shorter eating window. You might be used to eating smaller meals throughout the day instead of concentrating them during a specific period of time.

One of the consequences, especially if you follow the warrior diet or other similar plans, is that you can become too full and feel uncomfortable. That means that you can really have a hard time sticking to this diet because you suffer hunger and cravings during fast and you suffer from overeating during the eating time. Basically, if that happens, you are always uncomfortable.

This is one of the reasons why I've suggested more than once that you don't force yourself and always pay attention to how you feel.

However, if you really want to try the most extreme methods, at least eat as many nutrient-dense foods as you can, so that you are getting adequate nutrition without feeling sick.

Another downside, and this happens with many diets, is that you find yourself constantly thinking about food and eating and you obsess over eating and fasting windows.

This could also happen when you are with you friends and acquaintances. You might have to reschedule a night out if your friends are planning during your fast window.

Also, just because something works for you, that doesn't mean it also works for all your friends, family and colleagues. So keep your eating plans and health goals to yourself without trying to convince everybody else to follow it too. Even though you might have the best intentions and really want to help them, it won't be appreciated unless specifically asked.

It's really normal, when we find something that we like or that works for us, we immediately want to help everybody else. But this seldom works and often pushes people away.

Intermittent fasting is not meant to become an obsession. It is a way of training yourself to listen to your body and understand it better. By that I mean that it forces you to pay attention in order to tell when it is really hungry, when it is satisfied, when it feels energized and vital or when it feels tired, stressed or deprived.

This is an issue with many diets, they soon become obsessions and often fail. The only way to make it work is developing a healthy relationship first and foremost with yourself and your body. Then treat food as fuel not as entertainment or as a way to escape emotional issues.

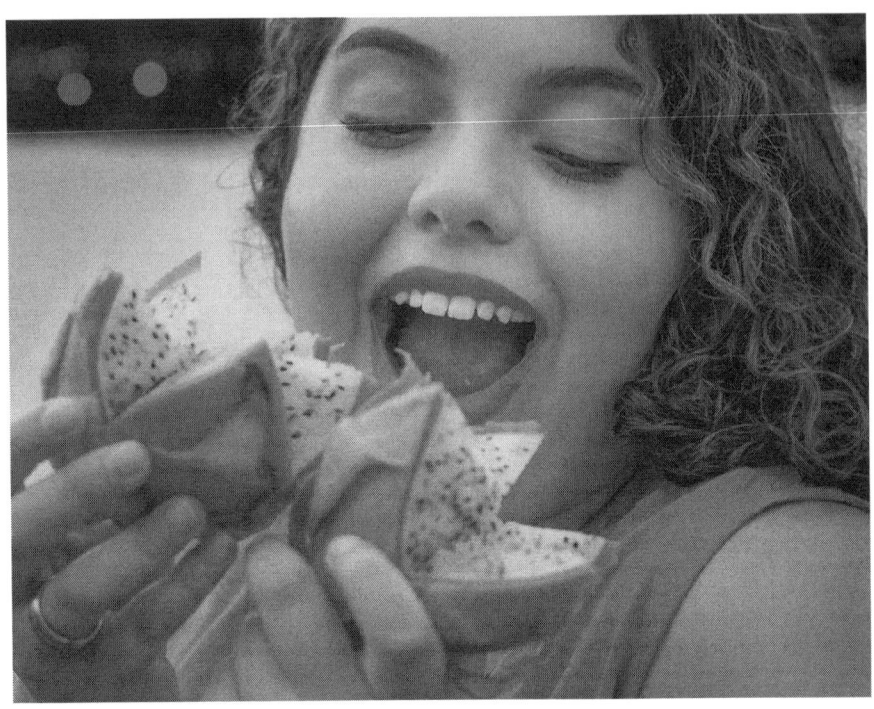

Some people wonder if it's possible to work out when fasting and there are some contradictory theories on this matter. However, there are many studies which support the theory that working out when fasting is possible and can also be beneficial. This applies to short period of fasting (like in the 16:8 method for example).

I suggest that you pay attention to how you feel and start making changes little by little. I also suggest that you talk to your doctor before starting a diet or exercise program.

Figuring out *when* to work out while on the intermittent fasting program is probably one of the most commonly asked questions. You can still do your regular workouts while intermittent fasting, you just might want to take it easy when you fast and choose more challenging activities during the eating window.

One of the downsides is reduced athletic ability, this might happen when you are fasting due to lack of energy and strength. As suggested, to bypass this issue you simply choose less intense activities during fasting periods.

The intensity of your workouts can make a big difference. Let's say you like yoga and HIIT training (high intensity interval training), you could choose yoga during fasting and HIIT sessions during the eating window.

If you do decide to workout when you are fasting, be careful with your cardio workouts. High-intensity cardio, like running or HIIT, can be a little hard on your body when you haven't been eating for a prolonged period of time. So simply make sure that you don't schedule your cardio workouts on days when you are fasting.

Many people who've been on an intermittent fasting diet suggest that you do your workouts shortly before you are going to start your eating phase. Of course, this may vary based on the type of workout you do, how you feel and how long you fast for.

If you are following the 16:8 then you might want to do cardio activities after you have entered the eating window, or at least allowing for a protein shake or a small healthy snack (some nuts for example) before starting the rigorous routine.

Some people who have extremely intense workout routines, like crossfit, find that they need a boost in protein and carbs prior to a workout. If this is the case, you may be someone who should do your workouts during your eating phase, and not your fasting phase.

Let's now look at *the benefits* of working out while on the intermittent fasting program. There are a number of reasons to schedule your workouts during fasted periods, as long as you aren't feeling sick or faint.

First of all, it helps your body get stronger and burn more fat. Exercising while fasting can also help with digestion. Many people find that eating shortly before or after a workout makes it harder to digest, leading to a variety of stomach problems.

Each person is different, each body is different and reacts in different ways to new eating and workout schedules. For this reason, it's really difficult to decide beforehand which method would be the best plan for you to follow.

As you can understand, the human body has amazing capabilities and it adapts to extreme situations.

Part III - Intermittent Fasting 16:8 Step by Step Guide

1

16:8 Method: How to Follow It

There is research available for this version of the intermittent fasting diet. Research has shown that this is an effective way to help people lose weight, lower their blood pressure, and reduce the risk of diabetes.

This method is a lot easier for most people to follow than other versions of the intermittent fasting diet that require 24 hours of fasting at a time if not up to 36 even.

By following the 16:8 method, you fast for 16 hours most of which is at night during sleep. In this 16-hour window there has to be no calorie intake. You can drink plenty of water, especially in the morning when you wake up, and some plain coffee or tea unsweetened.

During the 8-hour eating window make sure you follow a healthy and nutritious eating program. That isn't complicated and the benefits are well worth a try.

Scheduling your meals is pretty easy if you choose the 16:8 method. I've given a suggestion above (eating between 11.00 a.m. and 7.00 p.m.) based on what I believe to be the easiest way but that depends on your daily commitments and activities.

With that said, studies have shown that eating earlier at night is preferable than eating late and going to bed on a full stomach. So if, like in my example, you eat your last daily meal at 7.00 p.m. and you go to bed at 11.00 p.m. that's plenty of time between the meal and bedtime.

This does not mean that you have to do it that way. It really depends on your lifestyle. If you want to choose to eat between 8.00 a.m. and 4.00 p.m. that's fine too. Just pick an *8-hour eating window* and follow through no matter what others are doing (family, colleagues, friends…).

One thing that will make it easier for you to stick to a new healthy regimen is planning. That means that you reduce chances of ending up eating the first thing available (at the vending machine, drive through or whatever is left in your pantry).

If you exercise, you will need fuel to have sufficient energy to complete a workout program. Fuel means nutrients, good energy for your body. The more percentage there is of genuine and fresh food in your meals, the more likely you are to lose weight.

Whether you are fallowing the 16:8 method and fasting all night, or even if you are fasting two days a week, taking in high calorie foods during non-fast periods, or drinking any kind of beverage other than pure water, tea or black coffee, can ruin your weight-loss plans. That's because a lot of your calorie deficit is being compensated by extremely high calorie intake during the eating window and you won't be able to lose weight.

Since many times people eat out of boredom, keeping busy also helps. Watching TV induces hunger so try to reduce it to a minimum. If you keep yourself busy you will be able to keep the cravings at bay and actually enjoy the benefits of intermittent fasting. You could plan your fast on days when you are most busy so that you don't get time to obsess over your fast

Some of the basic problems that you might have to go through during the first period of fasting, such as the ones we've just mentioned (overcoming boredom and the tendency to think about food; anger and cravings) can be lessen by drinking plenty of water and unsweetened coffee or tea in moderation. Green tea is also an excellent remedy for food cravings.

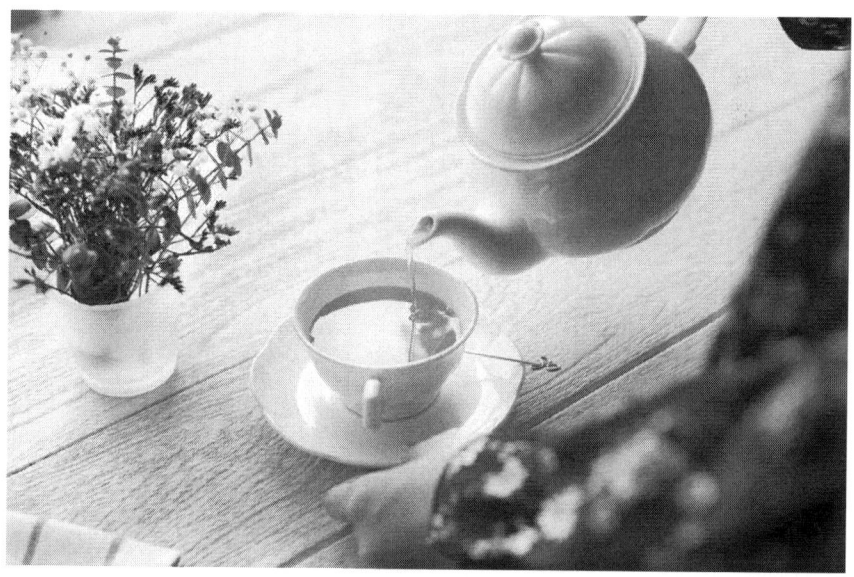

When it comes to beverages like coffee and tea, balance is always the key. Too much coffee can be harmful, a small amount can be beneficial.

High levels of caffeine may cause issues related to the adrenal glands and subsequently, have a detrimental impact on your health in the long run, particularly when it comes to adrenal malfunction which may lead to thyroid problems, insomnia, excessive fat build up, low immunity and fatigue apart from a number of other serious problems.

Choosing healthy fats (like fish, extra virgin olive oil and nuts); proteins (poultry; lean meat; eggs); complex carbs; fiber, vitamins, and minerals will also be very helpful, not only to normalize your body weight, but to lessen the effects of cravings, sugar crashes, fatigue and irritability.

If you are just starting out and you've never tried fasting before, I suggest you experiment and see what works for you. There are fasting that range from one day to two days per week. You could first try an hourly fast (like the 16-hour fast) before fasting for an entire day.

You can do a lunch-to-lunch or dinner-to-dinner fast, if you find it convenient or spread the fast over two days where you can sleep through more. However, I wouldn't suggest fasting for more than 24 hours.

Here are a few extra tips that you could adhere to when planning out your program.

If you are adopting the intermittent fasting plan to lose weight, you need to fit all your meals within your eating window.

Know your schedule, plan ahead. Intermittent fasting is mostly about timing and many people might tell you that it doesn't matter what food you eat during the eating window but, personally, I think *food does matter*. What you put into your body has a consequence not only on the way you look but most importantly on the way you feel.

This is an essential concept to understand for any kind of eating program to work. You might say: *"who cares anyway, a muffin or a cupcake is not going to make a difference on how I fit into my pants"* and this is focusing on the outer effect and it will soon lead to giving up because outer results take time to be visible. But how about how you *feel?* That is something you experience right away. How does a certain type of food make you feel? That is the question you want to ask yourself if you want to stick to your plans (and fit in your pants!).

With that said, it's true that your eating times and cut-off times are the cornerstones of intermittent fasting and you must comply with them for IF to be beneficial.

The fasting interval can last for eight to 36 hours.

Let's now take a look at the most important guideline about the fasting window, especially if you decide to fast for more than 16 hours. This phase is especially helpful for those needing to drop serious excess weight. As a good starting point, consider introducing a few hundred calories a day (during fast) instead of going 0 from the start. This can be adjusted as needed once your weight loss goals are met. Most intermittent fasting enthusiasts like to stay around this area to continue to reap the health benefits of fasting.

The key is to ensure that you maintain a stable feeding window time. The time and the type of food you eat, also could to be adjusted according to the plan for that day. If you are exercising, you will need more carbs than fats, to give you energy. We are talking healthy carbs here not simple sugar. Complex carbs like wholegrains, fruits and vegetables.

Similarly, on days when you are resting from physical activity, fats will be of more value. Healthy fats (think nuts, salmon, extra virgin olive oil, 100% natural nut butter like coconut or peanut butter).

Eat lots of whole, un-processed foods and ensure that you have good protein consumption every day (eggs, lean meat and seafood).

The important thing is to watch what you eat during days when you workout.

Many people who embark on Intermittent Fasting usually find that their lives are controlled by their eating windows and fasting windows. They need to constantly check the timing and plan things out. All these inconveniences can be avoided with proper planning.

Look at your schedule and preferences. What time do you wake up? What time is your lunch break at work? Do you prefer eating upon waking or would you rather go to sleep on a full stomach?

It is vital that you know your schedule and preferences. If you like going to bed with a full stomach, you'll probably have to schedule your eating window to start many hours after waking. What if you're at work and get hungry? Will you be able to take a break and eat your first meal when your eating window opens?

All these are considerations you must bear in mind when choosing which intermittent fasting method you want to adopt and then plan your fasting accordingly.

Now, just because the intermittent fasting 16:8 method is easy to understand and simple to plan, that doesn't mean it's also easy to apply. Especially because first you have to be very disciplined on your meal time and also because you still need to be mindful of what you eat and calorie intake.

If you are just starting out with this method, give yourself some time to adjust to the new routine. In case you "cheat" or for some reason you don't follow through in the way that you wish, don't think that you ruined it or you screwed up (again). All that will only make you feel miserable and it won't bring any good results.

Give yourself some time and if you fall off track just get back on track.

Here are the most common pitfalls you might want to avoid.

Indulging in too much junk food and sugar drinks as well as snacking late at night or after the 8-hour eating window.

If you are not losing weight, or if you are not reaping any benefits from the intermittent fasting 16:8 method, you might want to reduce those chips and ice cream snacks.

Another pitfall is being scared of hunger. That actually triggers thinking about food and consequently hunger. If you follow the 16:8 method, there is no reason for you to be scared of being hungry because you'll be eating almost regularly. Besides, if you reduce sugar (in all its many forms), eat plenty of fiber and protein your body will adjust and you won't feel the urge to eat all the time.

Focus on what you are doing moment by moment and have your desired end-results in mind. *Nothing worth having doesn't require effort.*

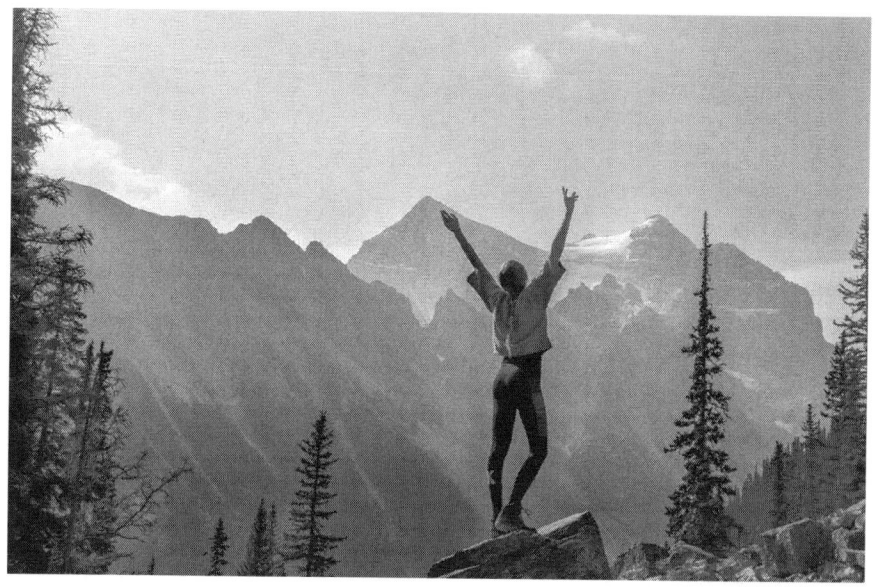

If you are eating clean on your eating period and still not losing weight, it likely means you are not moving your body enough. Exercise is essential not only for weight loss but for your overall health. Just because you are eating healthy and fasting for 16 hours straight, that doesn't mean that you will automatically get toned and fit. You need to pick some sort of fun activity to move your body, keep it flexible and vital.

It's tempting for some to slow down their activities because they are fasting but don't fall into this. Especially if you chose the 16:8

method. You will soon realize that exercise actually frees up more energy and you will want to be even more active throughout the day in all the things that you do. That will feel great.

If you follow the plan I've suggested (breakfast at 11.00 a.m. – lunch at 2.00 p.m. – small snack at 4.00 p.m. and dinner at 7.00 p.m.) you could workout for a half hour around noon or around 6.00 p.m. according to your schedule. Just make sure you workout safely and not immediately after a meal otherwise you might feel uncomfortable and have cramps.

If you are a beginner, I suggest that you avoid sharing your weight-loss goals and eating regimen with others who might discourage you. Sometimes sharing your plans with people who are not encouraging and supportive it's like throwing water on a spark before it can catch fire.

If you are planning a dinner with your friends or family, simply adjust your schedule for that day so that you can still fast for 16 hours. If they are eating very rich, calorie loaded foods just simply order a lighter meal and you don't have to explain or justify yourself for what you eat. If you really feel like you do, because maybe you usually eat the same kind of food, just say that you are not as hungry or that you ate too much at lunch or whatever comes up as needed. The explanation will come if you relax and don't make a big deal out of it. Besides I've learned that nobody really keeps track of me except me, and that is probably always the case with everyone.

Another trick I've learned is to pretend you are receiving a phone call. Excuse yourself for a minute and when you get back at the table just say that you are done and you are not hungry anymore. Again, don't make it look like a big deal and no one will notice.

This is an important concept because even if you don't realize it on a more conscious level, the people you surround yourself with have a huge impact on your behavior.

These were my special suggestions for you if you want to start a diet and more specifically if you have chosen the 16:8 method. Use them and I'm sure you will be fine; it just takes a little practice.

More on the 16:8 Intermittent Fasting Protocol. Following the 16:8 intermittent fasting program.

If there was one intermittent fasting method that most people tend to try first, it is probably the 16:8 protocol. This is mainly due to its simplicity.

I believe that this protocol is especially useful for *beginners* since you don't have to wait as long in between eating periods.

Many people struggle with intermittent fasting that requires going 24 hours or longer without eating. This is what is required when you follow the Warrior Diet or the Eat-Stop-Eat method of intermittent fasting.

With the 16:8 method, there are just a few hours in the morning and a few hours in the evening where you are not eating while awake.

As your body becomes accustomed to the new protocol less hunger will occur, and mostly it will occur when it's actually time to eat because the body will adapt to the new schedule.

If you like to go out at night, or if you are used to going out with friends in the evenings, you might be better off starting the fast window later, then skipping breakfast and eating a late lunch the following day.

The 16 hours of fasting might be difficult but only for the first few days.

2

Intermittent Fasting Delicious Meal Plan

Seven Fasting Breakfast Ideas

1. High Protein Smoothie

You can easily make a delicious and nutrient-dense high protein shake with avocado, almond milk (100% natural with no added sugar), fresh baby spinach leaves and protein powder.

With this smoothie you will feel full and satisfied because of the protein and the healthy fats in the avocado. Spinach will give you energy and a good fiber intake.

Note: all leafy green vegetables are filled with nutrients, make sure you consume plenty (spinach, kale, beets etc.)

If you prefer some other type of nut milk, that's fine as long as you pick the healthiest option which means the one that has less ingredients in it (read labels). You could buy 100% natural walnut milk or oat milk etc.

2. Fresh fruit platter

When you wake up, you've been fasting which means that, especially at the beginning of you journey with the intermittent fasting diet, your body will crave for rich foods filled with carbs. Donuts, bagels, muffins, pancakes and the like. If instead of giving in, you prepare a fresh fruit platter, you will do your body a great favor and it will reward you with vibrant energy.

Alternate depending on your taste, it could be an apple and a banana with cinnamon on top. Strawberries, blueberries and grapes. A peach some prunes and apricots. As long as it's fresh and with no added sugar.

You could drink a cup of unsweetened tea or plain coffee.

3. Veggie Omelet

To make this omelet have some veggies already cooked, it could be zucchini, spinach, carrots. Whisk a couple of eggs, add a pinch of salt and black pepper, your vegetables and cook on a hot pan with a teaspoon of butter or a drizzle of olive oil.

Note: if you use butter, make sure it's of good quality and preferably grass-fed. If you choose olive oil, make sure it's good quality, extra virgin olive oil.

Again, you could drink a cup of unsweetened tea or plain coffee.

4. Low fat Greek yogurt and nuts

When choosing what to eat, you want to avoid the type of food that causes cravings. That is sugar in all its many forms. Simple carbs, like baked products, it's basically sugar.

Instead you could try a fresh low-fat Greek yogurt with berries and nuts on top. If you like it, you can also add cinnamon and a teaspoon of raw honey on top.

5. Oatmeal

Buy fresh oats and cook it for a few minutes with a cup of hot water or half water and half of your favorite nut milk.

You can eat the oatmeal with fruits or nuts on top. Cinnamon and honey.

6. Hard boiled eggs and fresh spinach

I prefer room temperature boiled eggs so, personally, I cook them the day before. I like to sprinkle some cinnamon and black pepper on top of my hard-boiled eggs.

You can add fresh spinach leaves with natural raisins (no sugar, the plain kind). Or you can lightly sauté your spinach in a pan with a drizzle of extra virgin olive oil or a little grass-fed butter.

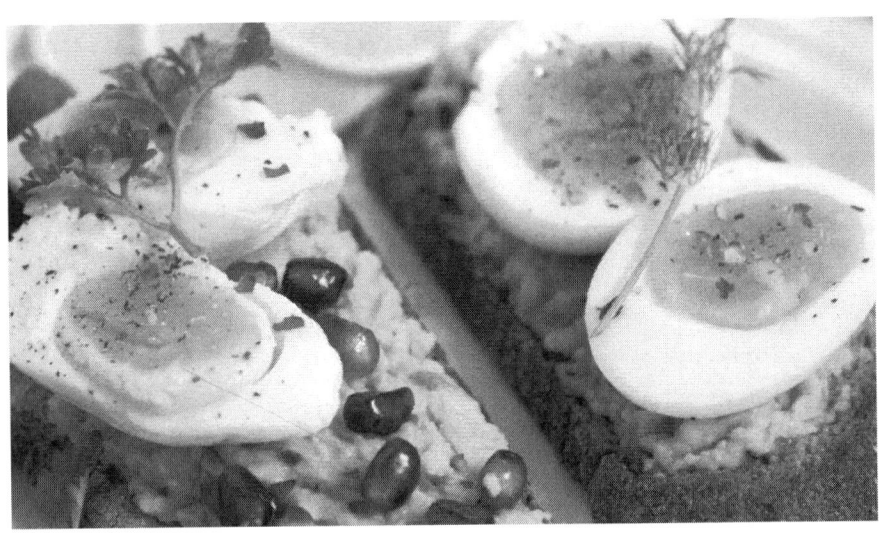

7. Whole grains cereal

A bowl of whole grains cereal and your favorite nut milk. I like to add some nuts or pecans to my cereal and nut milk.

Mix and match these 7 breakfast idea according to your taste and to what you have available. These kind of breakfast will give you energy and will nourish your body. At the beginning you might still crave for simple carbs but it's only temporary.

You can use these ideas for healthy snacks as well, maybe in smaller portions.

Seven Lunch Ideas

The thing with lunch is that many people are usually not at home during lunch. So if you are not used to preparing your food, you might think it's a problem to have it ready, heat it, store it etc. I assure you that it is not that hard, it's just a matter of habit and a little planning ahead. Beside, the simpler the better so carrying a banana or a hard-boiled egg is not a big deal. You can have some baby carrots with you or cut some celery and fennels and place them in a container.

Also, get yourself some containers that work in the freezer, fridge, and microwave. Then you can easily take healthy meals with you.

1. Romaine lettuce wraps

You can easily fill some large lettuce with tuna fish and tomatoes and prepare some delicious healthy wraps. You can add some fresh oregano or basil, a pinch of salt and pepper.

You can alternate lettuce with cabbage and you can replace tuna fish with feta cheese or chicken strips.

2. Broccoli salad

In a bowl, combine thin sliced broccoli and bell peppers, black olives and scallions. Whisk some apple cider vinegar and extra virgin olive oil. Add salt and pepper.

3. Cauliflower and lentil salad

Steam cauliflower florets for about 7 minutes, let cool and slice it. Cook lentils in boiling water for about 35 minutes and let cool. In a large bowl, mix together cauliflower and lentil, add raisins and season with the Mediterranean emulsion which is very simple to make: whisk the juice of a fresh squeezed lemon and a little extra virgin olive oil. Add salt and pepper to taste and enjoy!

4. Chicken and veggies

I suggest that you lightly sauté your vegetables in a pan with a drizzle of extra virgin olive oil, add salt and pepper. If you thin slice the vegetables it takes a shorter time for them to cook and they also cook more evenly.

Simply grill your chicken breasts and season with some fresh Mediterranean herbs like oregano or rosemary.

You can have this meal hot, with chicken and veggies on the side, or you can let cool everything then slice and mix together in a bowl or a container to take with you.

I assure you that, once you get used to this new method, you'll prepare these meals in less than 30 minutes.

5. Ground beef strips and veggies

Cook beef on a hot pan and then slice it into thin strips. Cook some green beans with extra virgin olive oil and half cup of hot water until all water is reduced and green beans are soft but not mushy.

Again, you can have this meal hot, with beef and veggies on the side, or you can let cool everything then slice and mix together in a bowl or a container to take with you.

6. Smoked salmon platter and arugula

Place smoked salmon on a platter (or a container if you have to take it with you). Add thin sliced avocado on top, pepper and fresh squeezed lemon juice. Eat the salmon with a side of arugula seasoned with the Mediterranean emulsion (whisk the juice of a fresh squeezed lemon and a little extra virgin olive oil) and few raisins.

7. Stuffed zucchini

Steam zucchini for about 3-5 minutes then cut it in halves and carefully empty the zucchini without breaking them in order to put the stuffing in. If the zucchini is too long, it might help to cut it in two pieces first then in halves and then empty it and then fill it with meat as follows.

Fill zucchini with minced meat. Add salt and pepper, a drizzle extra virgin olive oil and bake at 356 F for about 40 minutes.

You can alternate these meals and also you could use them as dinner ideas as well depending on your taste and what you have available.

Seven Dinner Ideas

These ideas might be helpful for you and your family to eat genuine foods and enjoy a healthy lifestyle. They are easy to make with simple ingredients and they taste really good.

Did you know that, once you start eating clean and you keep at it for a while then junk food will smell, look and taste disgusting for you?

That is exactly what happens. It is like people who smoke and then stop smoking, after a while they can't tolerate cigarette smell any longer.

1. Mediterranean style deviled eggs

Soak white beans (like cannellini beans) in hot water the night before you want to make this recipe. (They need to soak for about 6/8 hours), please don't buy canned, pre-cooked. It's not the same!

Cook beans in boiling water for about 40/50 minutes and let cool.

You need hard boiled eggs, let them cool then cut them in halves and empty them, keep the yolk for the mousse.

Use beans to make a mousse: blend beans with cooked egg yolk. Add tuna fish, fresh parsley, salt and pepper and one or two tablespoons of water.

Mix well and add a drizzle of extra virgin olive oil. Use this mousse to fill the eggs.

2. Veggie frittata

Cook spinach in a pan with a little butter for few minutes, add salt. Whisk two eggs with a pinch of salt and pepper. Add eggs to your spinach. Cook on both sides for about 3/4 minutes.

You can substitute spinach with your favorite kind of vegetables like green beans, broccoli, zucchini or kale.

3. Brown rice and veggies

You can enjoy some rice every now and then preferably brown rice of the best quality possible. Cook according to instructions on the package and top with sautéed veggies, grilled chicken or turkey.

4. Grilled Salmon and veggies

Add sesame seeds on top of salmon and cook it on the grill or on a hot pan. If you can, buy wild caught, fresh Alaskan salmon. Serve with a side of shredded cabbage, carrots, and radishes seasoned with the Mediterranean emulsion (whisk the juice of a fresh squeezed lemon and a little extra virgin olive oil).

5. Chicken and nut salad

This is a delicious salad that you can make with leftover chicken. Add thin sliced celery; fresh seedless grape; walnuts (or pecans). Season with salt and pepper; low fat Greek yogurt and a drizzle of organic raw honey.

6. Sweet potato (pureed) and chicken thighs

Boil sweet potatoes in hot water, mash and season with grass-fed butter; salt, pepper and cinnamon. Cook chicken thighs in a pan with garlic, extra virgin olive oil, curry, dried prunes (about 3 for each chicken thighs) and bay leaves. First lightly brown the thighs on each side then add about two cups of water. Cover with a lid and let cook until all water is reduced (usually about 50 minutes for three thighs).

6. Greek salad

I love Greek salad it is really fresh, filling and healthy. I like to make it with arugula, feta cheese, thin sliced onions, black olives, thin sliced tomatoes, thin sliced apple and few raisins. Season with the Mediterranean emulsion (whisk the juice of a fresh squeezed lemon and a little extra virgin olive oil), salt, pepper and fresh oregano.

You can eat with a slice of good quality, whole grain bread (fresh not packaged) with some extra virgin olive oil on top!

As you can see the recipes I've suggested contain protein, plenty of vegetables, some complex carbs and fewer simple carbohydrates. There is no real secret to being healthy.

I'd like to give you a few more recipes to mix and match.

1. Chia seeds smoothie

This can be easily made with your favorite choice of 100% natural nut milk; chia seeds; crushed ice; oats and a teaspoon of low-fat Greek yogurt. Add your favorite berry mix like blueberries and strawberries or cranberries and raspberries. If you are really hungry, add a small banana as well.

2. Green Beans, spring onions and garlic tofu

This is a great vegan recipe that can serve as lunch or dinner.

Steam the green beans for about 8 minutes (when you cook green beans, always make sure that they are soft but not mushy). Let the green beans cool.

Cook the tofu on a pan lightly greased with a drizzle of extra virgin olive oil. Cook until slightly golden. Sauté thin sliced spring onions, garlic and green beans for about 5 minutes. Mix with cubes of tofu, add a little apple cider vinegar, toss and serve.

3. Rosemary chicken and carrot

Start by preheating the oven to 400 F. Sauté garlic in a small frying pan with a drizzle of extra virgin olive oil until lightly golden. Add thin sliced carrots, chopped chicken and rosemary. Season with salt and hot chili pepper. Add a cup of water and let cook for about 30 minutes. You can serve this dish with a small serving of steamed Jasmin rice.

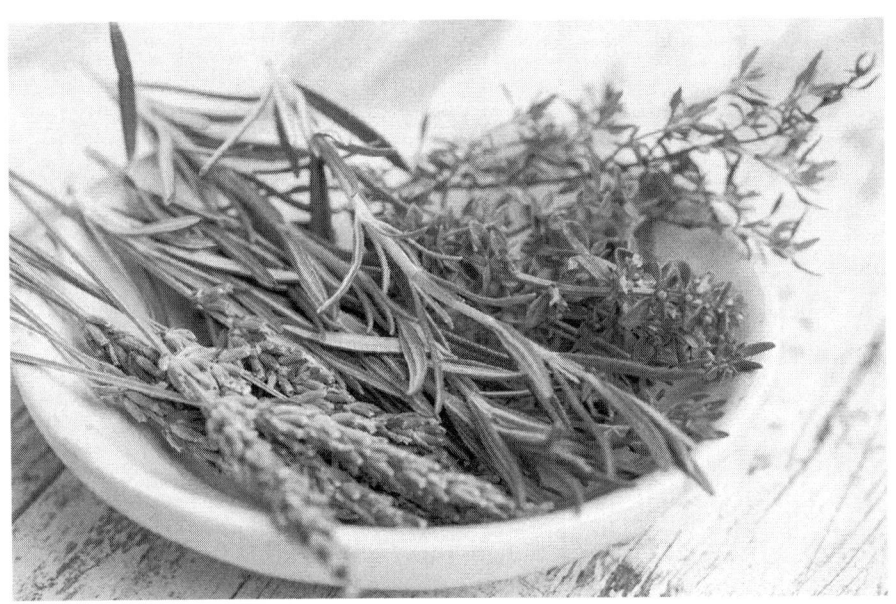

4. Cocoa and Raisin Cereal Bars

This is a sweet treat. It's healthy and it makes a perfect snack.

Preheat the oven at 356 F. Take a square cake tin pan and line with some greaseproof paper. In order to keep the oats from sticking to the greaseproof paper, grease with 1/2 teaspoon of butter. Soak raising in room temperature water for 10 minutes.

Mix oats, cocoa powder, coconut butter and drained raisins. If the mixture is too dry, add some coconut milk as well (100% natural with no added sugar). Bake for about 20 minutes depending on how much you are making. Make sure you don't overcook the mixture otherwise you bar will be too hard.

Once the mixture has cooked, remove from the tin so that you can cut it. Use a very sharp knife to cut perfect sized squares. Make sure that you allow the bars to cool before you pack them in an airtight container to refrigerate.

5. Grilled Portobello mushrooms

This recipe is very easy to prepare, it tasted good and has lots of nutrients. Preheat the oven at 356 F. Prepare the mushrooms, clean them thoroughly and cut them in small squares. Peal one or two potatoes and cut them in small pieces. Place mushrooms and potatoes on a baking tray, previously covered with baking paper, add garlic, rosemary, salt, pepper and a drizzle of extra virgin olive oil. Bake until thoroughly cooked (about 50 minutes) and enjoy.

6. Mediterranean scents mushrooms

Preheat the grill so that it is ready for the mushrooms. Clean mushrooms thoroughly and chop them finely into a small bowl. Add some garlic, olive oil and parsley to the chopped stalks. Now take a halved tomato and discard the seeds. Finely chop the tomato and add it to the stalks' mixture. Arrange the mushrooms on the grill and grill for around 3-4 minutes. Spread with tomato and garlic mixture. Season the mushrooms with salt and pepper and grill further for about 5 minutes. Your grilled mushrooms are ready to

Here are a few extra snack ideas that you will love.

Sabrina Smeraldini

1. Banana, apple, crushed ice and cinnamon smoothie.

2. Fresh peaches and a small amount of crushed Graham crackers on top.

3. Mixed nuts: almonds, walnuts, pecans and raisins.

4. Hummus, celery and carrot sticks.

5. Hard-boiled egg with apple and cinnamon on top.

6. Apple and 1 teaspoon of your favorite 100% natural nut butter.

7. 1 tablespoon of coconut butter, 100% plain and natural.

3

Adequate Hydration

Water is the most precious thing for the body and it helps to keep it hydrated, cleanse itself, reduce brain fog and fatigue and consequently make you feel better and more vital.

Make sure you stay hydrated. Whether you are a fasting expert or if you have never fasted before, I cannot stress enough the importance of staying hydrated.

When your body detoxes, on your fasting days, and starts releasing some of the toxins it has built up in years of junk food eating and drinking, it will go much smoother if you are drinking a proper amount of natural water.

If you don't drink enough, not only can you experience fatigue and brain fog - even in their most acute forms such as lethargy and weakness - but also stomach pains, along with other unpleasant symptoms of dehydration. And this is true regardless of your diet plan.

Also, be mindful of the fact that often, what you perceive as hunger, is actually dehydration. You might be really thirsty and need a large glass of fresh, pure, clear water.

Always make sure that you drink plenty of pure, natural water to cleanse your body and your mind as well (you know… Hydration helps with brain-fog issues and fatigue). Please don't think that drinking lots of soda helps you with hydration, even if it's diet soda, the same goes for wine and beer. When I speak of hydration I'm referring to H2O pure and simple. Ok?

Also, avoid or reduce alcohol intake since it contains lots of sugar and calories. Not only that, alcohol weakens your will power and so increase chances of you giving up on your fasting or allowing yourself some comfort food (aka hyper-calorie-junk).

One of the most frequently asked questions about the Intermittent Fasting Diet is whether coffee and tea are allowed during the fasting period. The idea of the Intermittent Fasting Diet is to avoid any calorie intake during fasting. For this reason, coffee and tea are permitted only when consumed plain (no sugar and no dairy added).

With that said, if you are used to drinking coffee or tea with a lot of sugar or cream, it might take a little while for you to get used to plain black. Try reducing sugar and cream gradually as you begin until you reach the point where you are ok with plain black. If you do this, I assure you that you'll be reaching a point where you actually don't want sugar and cream any longer. This is because your taste buds will get used to the new version.

Drinking lots of water, some coffee or tea will help you feel less hungry during fasting periods.

Proper hydration is crucial at all times, whether you're fasting or not.

4

Intermittent Fasting: The Easy Strategy (Extra Info & Tips)

As we've seen, there are various Intermittent Fasting protocols available, and each has different rules. Some dieters choose to fast for 12 to 16 hours. Others plan a 72-hour fast.

While it's true that there are various intermittent fasting methods, basically there are two main approaches. The first is alternating eating days with fasting days. The second variant is what you will see in intermittent fasting diets like the 5:2 Diet. This requires you to eat regularly five days and fast for two days.

Much of the information I've provided about the intermittent fasting diet works well with all methods. Some people prefer the first approach for long term results in terms of weight loss as well as ease of use and likelihood of being able to stick with the program.

Another method sometimes mentioned is the "Fat Loss Forever". Pretty cool name right? Just by saying it you can picture beautiful slender bodies full of energy and vitality. It definitely attracts the attention of people who would like to shed some pounds.

It is considered as some kind of an integration of the best of the 16:8, eat stop eat and the warrior diet.

The Fat Loss Forever diet offers a structured 7-day schedule that helps the body get used to fasting. This plan allows one "cheat day" after which you are required to fast for 36 hours. It's a specific plan and it can be a bit difficult to stick to it (I mean, 36 hours!). The seven-day cycle is then segmented to accommodate the various fasting protocols. It is better to save the longest fasts for the days when you are the busiest. This helps getting your mind off food and focus on your activities.

This diet is ideal for those who really love cheat days and do not want to give them up.

The Eat Stop Eat plan requires you to fast for 24 hours either once or twice per week. During the 24 hour fasting you can drink water, plain coffee or tea but you are not allowed to eat.

You can go back to eating regularly once the fasting period has finished. In order to make the most of the Eat Stop Eat intermittent fasting diet, it is important to incorporate frequent workouts as well as resistance training. This diet is ideal for all the dedicated healthy food lovers that are looking for a boost in their lifestyle.

This is a flexible diet program and you can adjust the fasting phase according to how well your body responds. Take it easy at the beginning and increase the fasting time as your body gets used to it.

The main challenge of the Eat Stop Eat plan is that 24 hours without any calories can be tough and can lead to headaches and fatigue.

In the Warrior Diet you are supposed to fast for around 20 hours each day; so that the day will end with one large meal. The effectiveness of the warrior diet is dependent on the type of food in the large meal.

During the fasting phase of the diet, you can have fresh squeezed juice (don't drink common bottled fruit juice because they are often filled with sugar, preservatives and dyes) small servings of protein, vegetables and raw fruits. Eating will occur in the four hours that are left at night. It is advised to have vegetables first and then have proteins and fat. Carbohydrates should be the last option when you still need to eat more.

Personally, I am not a fan of eating one large meal at the end of the day. However, some people find it helpful that you are not completely fasting during the fasting period and can still have small portion of healthy foods.

This is also another reason why I personally am not a fan of this method. Fasting is fasting, if you are eating is not fasting.

There are people who like to eat at night, maybe watching TV, and that's fine. Some will find this the perfect program to follow and reap benefits from it.

Another name for the alternate-day fasting is the Up-Day Down-Day. Some people consider it the easiest method, although you may have guessed by now that it really depends on personal preferences and individual needs.

This method consists of eating a very little amount of food one day and then eating regularly the next day.

The rule is that on the low-calorie days you use up to one fifth of the general calorie intake that you consume. So, let's say that women are allowed 2000 calories and men 2500 calories (and notice that this is a very generic rule. Calorie intake is to be calculated by taking into consideration many factors like age, height, level of activity, BMI – which stands for body mass index – and so on), then a fasting day would require 400 to 500 calories.

Down days are your fasting windows. I would suggest you work out on the up day, days when you are not fasting, since it can make it difficult to manage the fast if you are using up your energy for physical activity.

This diet is ideal for those who have a specific weight-loss goal in mind. If your level of self-discipline is high, you can manage this diet fairly easily. However, many people experience binge eating on days when they are not fasting.

Some athletes drink protein shakes on fasting days. However, since intermittent fasting preserves lean muscle, there's no need to take supplements.

Intermittent fasting works best when combined with strength training and high-intensity exercise, such as HIIT. Most gym goers claim that they are able to work out harder for longer while in on this program. Due to its beneficial effects on testosterone and growth hormone levels, the alternating fasting periods boosts your performance and overall strength. Working out will speed up your progress and maximize the effects of fasting.

Do not complicate things. Intermittent fasting is supposed to simplify your life not the other way around. Don't stress over calories, macros, or meal timing. Unless you have a specific need, there's no point in worrying about these things.

For the average person, meal timing and macro ratios make little difference. *Focus on eating clean and staying active.* This is the only effective key. No secret and no mystery.

If you have a hard time fasting, keep yourself distracted. Try yoga or Pilates, go out for a walk, drink herbal tea or get more sleep. If you stick to this plan long enough, your eating habits will improve significantly.

Final Thoughts

The body is a complex and sophisticated system that needs proper nutrients in order to work efficiently. These days we are faced with a constant onslaught of tempting junk food and non-nutritious, addictive snacks. Food has become some sort of entertainment.

At the same time, we lead more sedentary lives, made easier by technology and other devices to do things for us. Consequently, our level of physical activity has decreased to alarming levels.

Even shopping now it's mostly done online. If we so choose, we don't even have to walk in the mall or in the grocery store. We could virtually do everything just by sitting somewhere with internet connection.

The result is an increase in obesity and laziness and a loss in terms of recognizing the benefits of genuine ingredients and a much simpler life.

Many, if not the majority of health problems could be avoided with proper nutrition and a healthier lifestyle. Spending time outdoors instead of facing the screen all day would certainly help.

Our ancestors, as we've seen, had very different habits and obesity was not really a problem back then. They were used to being more active and eating less. Their body had both strength and stamina to withstand the worst conditions including prolonged hunger.

The intermittent fasting diet – if followed correctly - is one of the ways in which we can enjoy the benefits of healthy living.

In this book we have highlighted a number of ways to overcome your fears and given you many hints to adapt to fasting. Remember though it's all about effort, progress and consistency. And that is true regardless of what goal you want to achieve.

Besides, we've delved a bit more deeply in the 16:8 method but you can still explore all other methods as well. One of the advantages of the intermittent fasting diet is that you can really create it tailor-made for you, according to your needs.

Fasting is one of the easiest ways and it will allow you to choose freely from a number of healthy food options. You can select any number of recipes from this book and make a suitable diet plan.

Also remember, to align your fasting with some exercise routine, be it as simple as running. Working out will increase your metabolic rate, especially fat oxidation. Complementing your dieting routine with exercise will allow you to achieve your goals in a considerably shorter time.

Moreover, while you are fasting and watching your calories, resist the temptations of junk food. It might be difficult at parties and with friends, but try to schedule your weekday in a way that you can stick to your plans without renouncing your social life.

If you find that things are getting too stressful, make some changes to your plan, don't be too rigid. If you stop for whatever reason, don't be scolding yourself, start again. The whole point is to increase the quality of your life and feel better within and without.

As we've said at the beginning of this book, keep the goal in mind and remind yourself of the benefits of intermittent fasting. We've seen different ones such as prevention of many health problems and anti-aging.

With the given knowledge and information and a positive approach, there is no reason that you will not be able to achieve your goals whether it be weight loss, muscle gain or overall improved health.

~ ♣ ~

Please keep in mind that I am not a doctor and I am not a physician. I am passionate about food and healthy eating so what I write is personal knowledge based on my experiences. I enjoy sharing content and tips that I believe might be helpful for anyone who's interested in living a healthier lifestyle and feel better. So I really hope you enjoyed my book but I encourage you to consult your physician before starting a diet or an exercise program.

~ ♣ ~

CONCLUSION

~ ♣ ~

Did you enjoy this book?

I would love it if you could write your review. That would be really helpful for others who may be interested and benefit from the content I've shared.

If you would like to give me some suggestions, you can contact me at: infosmeraldini@gmail.com

Check-out my family's healthy appetizers recipes. From my Grandma's kitchen, in Tuscany, to your dinner table!

https://www.italianstylerecipe.net/easy-appetizers-gift/

Sincerely!

Sabrina Smeraldini

ABOUT THE AUTHOR

~ ♣ ~

Thank you for your interest in this book by Sabrina Smeraldini.

Sabrina Smeraldini grew up in Tuscany with her Italian Grandma, *Nonna Maria*, who inspired her to write about food, cooking and diets.

She has written various books on different diets including the Mediterranean Diet to promote the benefits of healthy eating.

She is founder of *italianstylerecipe.net* a site designed to share the love for cooking delicious and traditional recipes from Grandma's kitchen.

Sabrina's work is an encouragement to explore a new way of approaching food and experiencing the pleasure of going back to savoring natural, genuine meals. *Eating healthy is a lifestyle.*

~ ♣ ~

You can find Sabrina's books at the following link:

https://www.amazon.com/author/sabrinasmeraldini

Sabrina Smeraldini

Thank you!

Sabrina Smeraldini

@ Copyright di Sabrina Smeraldini

http://www.italianstylerecipe.net/

Printed in Great Britain
by Amazon